SURVIVING SYPHILIS

Beginners Comprehensive Approach To Combating & Managing Syphilis Outbreak Effectively

Nuel Nenji

Table of Contents

Introduction

The bacterium Treponema pallidum is responsible for causing syphilis, a type of STI. In extremely rare cases, syphilis can be spread through non-sexual contact with syphilis sores or when a woman transmits the disease to her child during pregnancy or childbirth. Syphilis progresses through distinct phases, each of which can cause serious health problems if left untreated. Here are the steps:

• Primary syphilis is the earliest stage of the disease and is characterized by the development of a chancre, a painless sore or ulcer, near the entry point of the bacteria. The genitalia, anus, and oral cavity are common locations for chancres to manifest. It's possible that the wound won't bother you anymore if the infection isn't addressed.

• Syphilis develops into its more serious secondary form if the initial infection is not successfully treated. Rash, oral sores, fever, exhaustion, and enlarged lymph nodes are all possible symptoms. These symptoms may come and go, but they can be very severe when they do appear.

• If syphilis is not treated during the secondary stage, it will progress to the asymptomatic latent stage. The illness has not been eradicated and could lie latent for years.

• Damage to the heart, brain, nerves, eyes, and blood vessels can occur in the later stages of syphilis, known as tertiary syphilis, if the infection is left untreated for a long period of time. Tertiary syphilis is potentially fatal and is associated with severe consequences.

The health risks associated with untreated syphilis are substantial. Penicillin or other antibiotics like doxycycline or azithromycin may be necessary, however curing the illness is possible at any stage. If you have engaged in unprotected sexual activity or come into touch with someone who has syphilis, it is imperative that you seek medical assistance and get tested if you suspect you have syphilis.

Complications and the spread of the disease can be avoided via prompt diagnosis and treatment. Syphilis and other sexually transmitted infections (STIs) can be avoided via the use of condoms and other safe sexual practices.

CHAPTER ONE
Transmission Methods

Direct contacts with infectious sores or the exchange of bodily fluids are the two most common ways for syphilis to spread. Here are the most common ways that syphilis is spread:

• Vaginal, anal, and oral intercourse are the most prevalent routes of syphilis transmission, although other forms of sexual contact can be a risk. The syphilis sore (chancre) or rash of an infected person can spread to their sexual partner by contact with the mucous membranes or torn skin. Syphilis can be spread between people of any sexual orientation or gender.

• Syphilis can be passed from an infected mother to her unborn child during pregnancy or delivery (a process known as "vertical transmission"). Consequences for the unborn child include stillbirth, preterm delivery, low birth weight, and various birth abnormalities; this condition is known as congenital syphilis.

• Although it is uncommon, syphilis can also be spread through non-sexual contact with a person who has syphilis lesions. This can happen when one person kisses another who has open sores, or when two people share a towel, razor, or needle that has been contaminated by the sick person. But syphilis is typically associated with sexual contact.

• There is no risk of contracting syphilis via shaking hands, hugging, or sharing a locker room or pool with someone who has the disease. Treponema pallidum, the bacterium responsible for syphilis, is not very hardy and dies off quickly when exposed to conditions outside of a human host.

Safe sex practices include always and properly using condoms, getting regular examinations for sexual health, and getting medical help right away if you think you have syphilis or have been in close contact with someone who does. To avoid having a baby born with syphilis, pregnant mothers should get prenatal care and be screened for the disease.

How To Recognize And Treat Syphilis

The symptoms of syphilis can be quite diverse, and they change as the illness progresses. Some patients with syphilis, especially in the early stages, may not show any symptoms at all. Each stage of the disease's development is marked by its own unique set of symptoms:

1. Initial Stage Syphilis:

• A chancre, a painless, round, and firm sore or ulcer, is the earliest symptom of primary syphilis.

• Genital, anus, and oral sites of infection are common entry points for chancroid bacteria.

• Because it causes little discomfort and can heal without medical intervention, a chancre often goes undiagnosed.

2. Syphilis secondary:

• Secondary syphilis can occur if the primary syphilis infection is not properly managed.

• Rash, mouth sores, fever, exhaustion, swollen lymph nodes, and muscle aches are all possible signs.

• The palms of the hands and the soles of the feet may break out in a rash.

• The severity of symptoms may increase from the initial stage.

3. Subclinical Syphilis:

• After the secondary stage, syphilis can go into a dormant phase in which no outward symptoms are present. A period of years may pass.

• Latent syphilis is an infection that is still present in the body and can develop into tertiary syphilis if not treated.

4. Syphilis, Tertiary Form:

• Years after the initial infection, tertiary syphilis can manifest and cause significant organ damage.

• Cardiovascular issues (like aortic aneurysms), neurological issues (like paralysis and dementia), and gummas (soft, non-cancerous growths) are all possible manifestations.

Warning: tertiary syphilis can be fatal.

Syphilis is usually diagnosed by a combination of the following methods:

1. A doctor or nurse will look over your medical history and evaluate any cuts, rashes, or other symptoms you may be experiencing.

2. The most common method of diagnosing syphilis is by a blood test. Common syphilis blood tests include:

• Venereal Disease Testing by the VDRL

• The RPR Test (Rapid Plasma Reagin).

• Test for Treponema pallidum (TPPA) particle agglutination.

• Antibodies produced by the body in reaction to a syphilis infection are what these tests look for.

3. Syphilis sore fluid samples can sometimes be studied using darkfield microscopy to see the Treponema pallidum bacteria up close and personal.

If you have engaged in unprotected sexual activity or come into touch with someone who has syphilis, it is imperative that you seek medical assistance and get tested if you suspect you have syphilis. In order to properly heal the illness and prevent consequences, early detection is essential, as is treatment with antibiotics, often penicillin.

In order to stop the spread of syphilis, the sexual partners of people who have tested positive for the disease should be checked as well. Sexually active people should get checked for STDs like syphilis and other sexually transmitted diseases on a regular basis.

CHAPTER TWO
Cure For Syphilis

The infection caused by syphilis can be treated with antibiotics. Antibiotics and their duration of use are determined by the severity of syphilis as well as other factors unique to the patient. Antibiotics typically prescribed for syphilis treatment are as follows:

• Antibiotics that contain penicillin are the best option for treating syphilis. Depending on the severity of the infection, the type and amount of penicillin prescribed will change.

One injection of penicillin is usually all that's needed to cure primary, secondary, and early latent syphilis. Benzathine penicillin G (Bicillin L-A) is the most popular kind.

Injections of penicillin are given repeatedly over a longer length of time to treat late-stage syphilis, including latent and tertiary.

• When penicillin is not an option owing to an allergy or another medical condition, doxycycline or tetracycline may be recommended as an alternative. Antibiotics like these are typically prescribed for longer periods of time than penicillin.

• Azithromycin: It may be utilized in some circumstances, especially for people who are allergic to both penicillin and tetracycline drugs. To treat syphilis in its early stages, a single dose is usually sufficient.

To guarantee comprehensive treatment of the illness, it is essential to take all of the medications your doctor prescribes. Verifying the treatment's efficacy with follow-up examinations is also crucial.

Sexual abstinence is recommended during syphilis treatment and until a healthcare physician says it is safe to resume. Notifying sexual partners and encouraging them to get tested and, if necessary, treated is also recommended for preventing further spread.

Treatment with penicillin is also necessary to prevent difficulties in newborns in cases of congenital syphilis (when a pregnant woman with syphilis transmits it to her baby).

In order to track the effectiveness of therapy and rule out any lasting side effects or consequences, syphilis patients should schedule follow-up appointments with their doctors on a regular basis.

If you have had recent contact with an infected person or think you may have syphilis, you should visit a doctor immediately. Curing the infection and halting its progression to more serious stages of the disease both depend on prompt diagnosis and treatment.

Reduction And Management

Public health measures and personal hygiene practices both play a role in preventing and controlling syphilis. Key preventative and control methods include:

1. Appropriate Sexual Behaviors:

• Always and properly use condoms when engaging in sexual activity, including oral, anal, and genital sex.

• Reduce the amount of sexual partners you have and pick ones who have had syphilis and other STI tests.

• Safe sex practices are crucial since syphilis can be passed on even in the absence of symptoms.

2. Testing & Screening Schedules:

• Regular STI screens, including for syphilis, are recommended for all sexually active people, but especially those who have more than one sexual partner or who engage in other high-risk sexual practices.

• Congenital syphilis can be avoided if pregnant women are tested for the disease early in their pregnancies.

3. Care and Informing Your Partner:

• If you have had contact with someone who has syphilis or if you think you might have syphilis yourself, see a doctor very away.

• If you have syphilis and have had sexual partners, you must let them know so that they can be tested and treated if necessary.

4. Preventing Congenital Syphilis

• Pregnant women should be screened for syphilis and given treatment if necessary to reduce the risk of the disease being passed on to their unborn children.

• The chance of having a child born with syphilis can be greatly reduced if the disease is diagnosed and treated early in pregnancy.

5. Tracking the State of Public Health:

• Syphilis cases should be reported to public health authorities by health departments and healthcare practitioners.

• Timely reporting is crucial for detecting epidemics and enforcing control measures.

6. Partner Support:

• When someone is diagnosed with syphilis, public health organizations may offer partner services to notify and test potential sexual partners.

• Partner services can aid in identifying and treating sick individuals, which can help curb the disease's spread.

7. Knowledge and understanding:

• Publicize the dangers of syphilis and other sexually transmitted infections through awareness campaigns and instructional initiatives.

• Stress the significance of encouraging frequent testing, early diagnosis, and safe sexual behavior.

8. Availability of Medical Care:

• Make sure people can afford and easily gain access to healthcare options like STI screening and treatment.

• Cost, stigma, and a lack of knowledge are just some of the barriers to healthcare that need to be addressed.

9. PrEP, or pre-exposure prophylaxis:

• PrEP is generally employed as an HIV preventative measure. HIV and syphilis have many of the same risk factors for transmission, therefore this may have a beneficial side effect of reducing the spread of syphilis. If you are at risk for HIV, talk to your doctor about pre-exposure prophylaxis (PrEP).

10. Study and Keeping Tabs:

• Improving syphilis prevention and control initiatives requires further study of the disease's epidemiology, drug resistance, and therapeutic alternatives.

• Healthcare practitioners, public health agencies, community organizations, and ordinary citizens must all work together to prevent and control syphilis. Syphilis and its sequelae can be reduced via early diagnosis and treatment, as well as through continued education and preventive initiatives.

CHAPTER THREE
Considerations Of Society And The Mind

Syphilis, like other STIs, can have serious implications for a person's social and psychological health, as well as their connections with others and their general happiness and well-being. Some of the psychological and social effects of syphilis are as follows:

• Syphilis, like other sexually transmitted infections (STIs), is often met with shame and stigma. The stigma associated with a syphilis diagnosis can have a devastating effect on a person's sense of worth and well-being.

• The diagnosis of syphilis can put a burden on any type of intimate relationship. It can be tough to tell a spouse you have HIV since it might cause trust issues, fights, or even the end of the relationship.

• Anxiety, depression, and other mental health issues may arise when a person with syphilis deals with the diagnosis and its repercussions. When dealing with complications or advanced stages of syphilis, the emotional toll can be devastating.

• The diagnosis of syphilis may prompt a person to alter their sexual habits. Others may have trouble with sexual intimacy and desire, while some may become more cautious and embrace safer sex practices.

• Notifying sexual partners of a syphilis diagnosis can be an emotionally taxing task, but it is also a legal requirement. The risk of spreading the disease may be higher if people are reluctant to tell their partners due to concerns about being judged or rejected.

• Barriers to Healthcare Some people may not be able to get the syphilis testing, treatment, and follow-up care they need because of things like a lack of health insurance, high out-of-pocket costs, or their location. These obstacles may cause a delay in diagnosis and treatment.

• Women infected with syphilis during pregnancy may worry about the effects of the disease on their unborn child. Concern about congenital syphilis is reasonable.

• The social and mental toll of syphilis can be lessened via the implementation of effective prevention and education initiatives. When people have access to reliable information about sexual health issues, they are better able to make educated decisions regarding prevention, testing, and treatment.

• Counseling and support groups can be quite useful in helping people with syphilis deal with the psychological and emotional effects of the disease. Counseling can help with the emotional difficulties, as well as with relationship and sexual health management techniques.

Syphilis, like other sexually transmitted infections (STIs), is a medical condition, and those who have been diagnosed with syphilis should not be condemned or ostracized because of it. The social and psychological effects of syphilis can be lessened via open and nonjudgmental discussion of sexual health, routine STI testing, and access to healthcare services. Better sexual health and well-being for affected individuals can also result from destigmatizing dialogues about STIs and fostering a culture of understanding and support.

Conclusion

Syphilis, in conclusion, is a STI brought on by the bacterium Treponema pallidum. It has different symptoms at different stages and can cause different problems if left untreated. Curing syphilis and keeping it from progressing to more severe stages requires prompt diagnosis and treatment with medicines like penicillin.

Individual behavior modification and community-wide preventative measures are both essential for syphilis management. Reducing the spread of syphilis requires safe sexual practices, regular STI testing, and appropriate treatment.

Overall sexual health and well-being can benefit from initiatives to lower stigma, increase knowledge, and spread support and education.

The social and psychological effects of syphilis include discrimination, difficulties in interpersonal relationships, and negative effects on psychological well-being.

Syphilis and other sexually transmitted infections (STIs) should be treated with compassion and understanding, with victims receiving assistance and open, nonjudgmental dialogue about sexual health being encouraged.

Syphilis is a very dangerous but curable disease. The negative effects of syphilis can be mitigated through a mix of preventative strategies, early diagnosis, and effective treatment. Key components of preventing and managing syphilis and other STIs include regular healthcare check-ups,

safe sexual behaviors, and informed
decision-making about sexual health.

THE END